the Plaque Pixie's

ORAL HYGIENE LESSON

by Richard Schmidt

COPYRIGHT

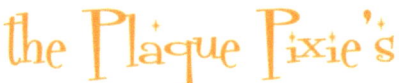

ORAL HYGIENE LESSON

Printed in the United States of America

First Printing, 2015

ISBN   978-1-508400-27-1

PLAQUE PIXIE BOOKS
Randolph, NJ 07869
www.plaquepixiebooks.com

Acknowledgements

RICHARD SCHMIDT

The people who have had the greatest impact on my life and me to dream:

My parents, Dr. Robert and Rebecca Giaquinta, without who has given me the education, inspiration, and encouragement to write these books.

Hysson Monia, who has been critical, in helping provide content and structure, as well as amazing support for my efforts.

All my teachers, colleagues, patients, and friends past and present, your contribution to my life and subsequently this book have been immense.

Finally the children, for whom all this matters, I hope that these books may make a positive impact in your lives.

"How you speak to your children becomes their inner voice...."

Anonymous
Wednesday - Aug 22, 2012 9:09 am)

the Plaque Pixie's

ORAL HYGIENE LESSON

by Richard Schmidt

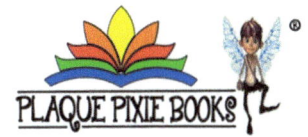

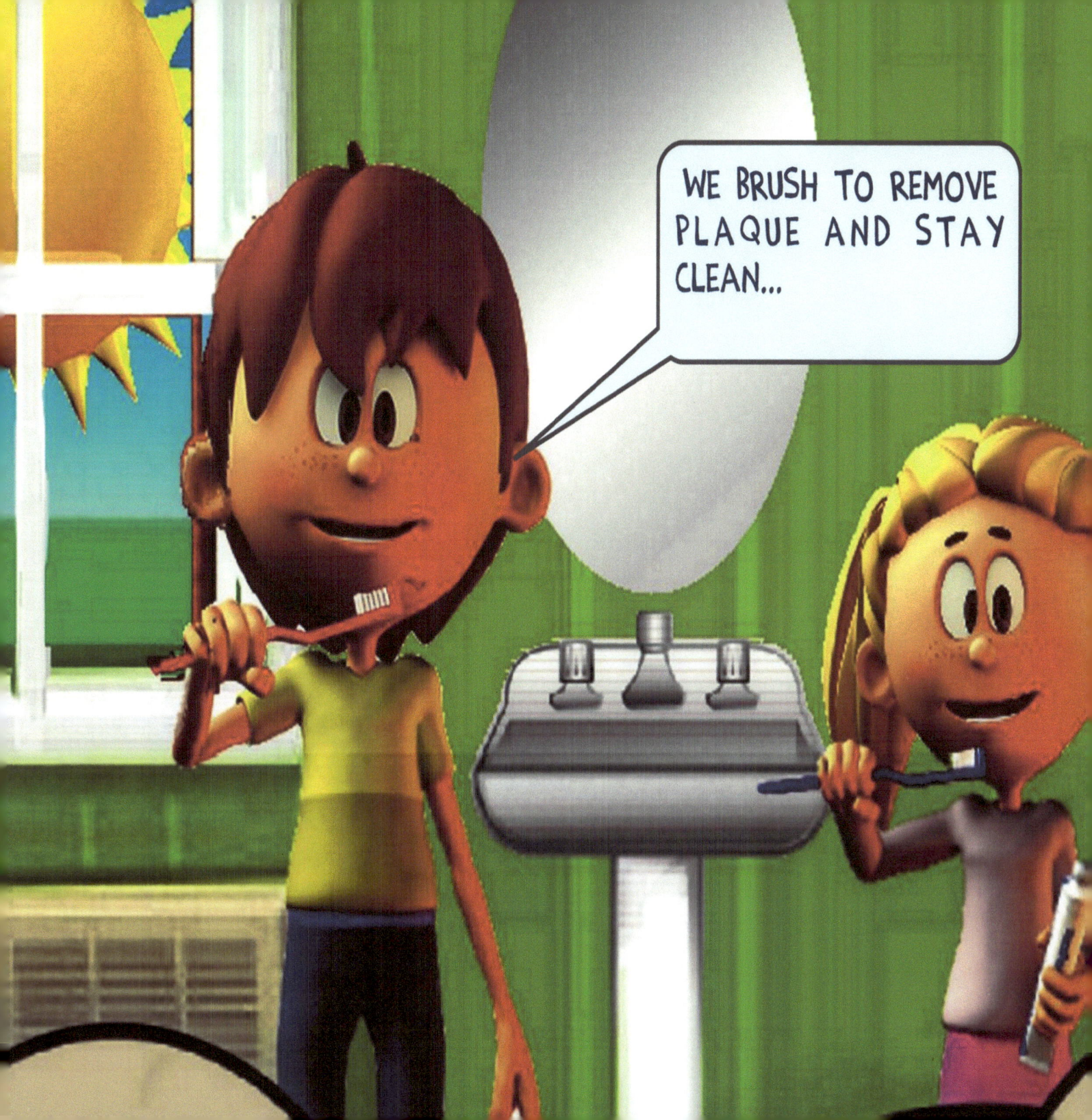

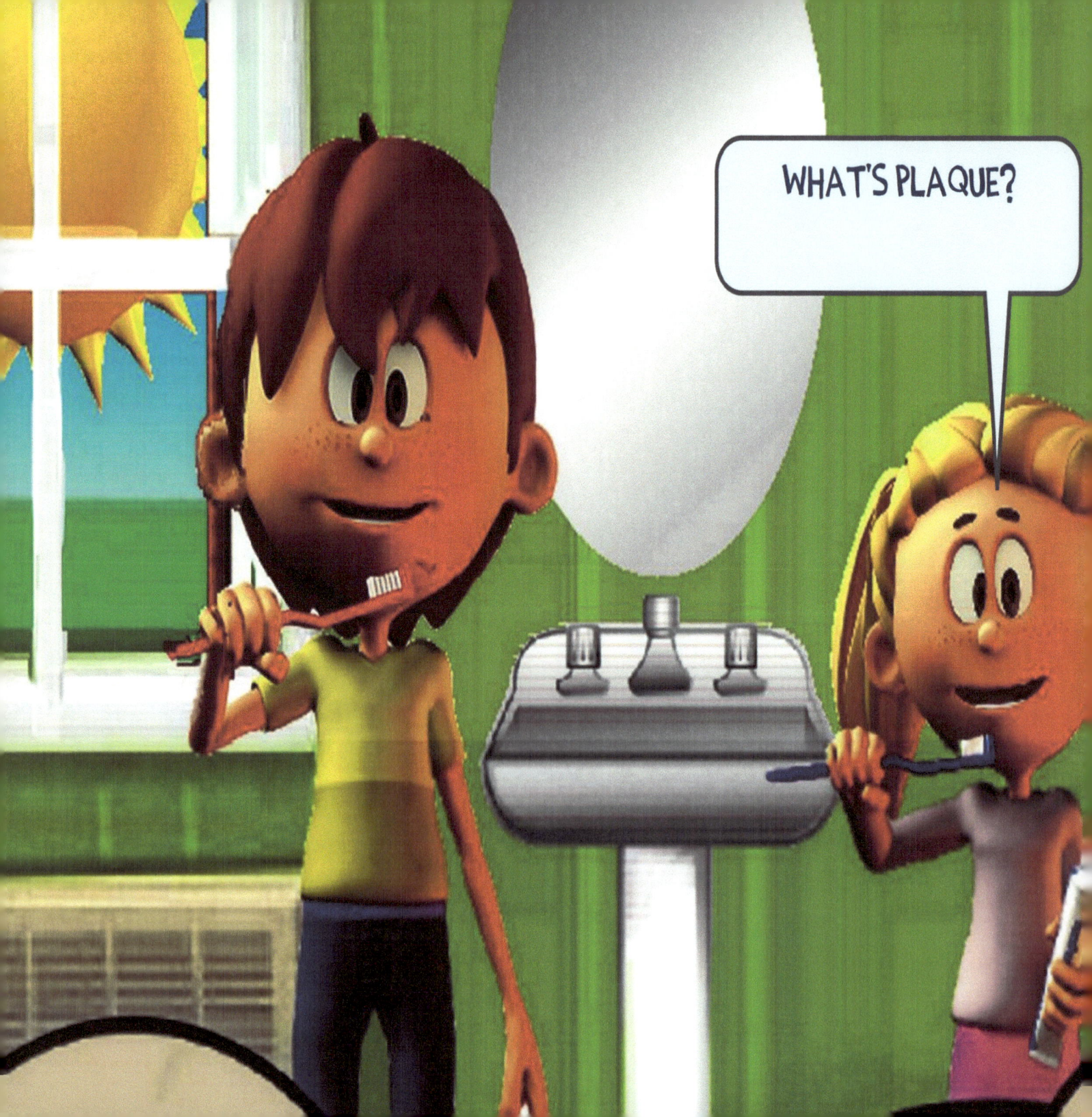

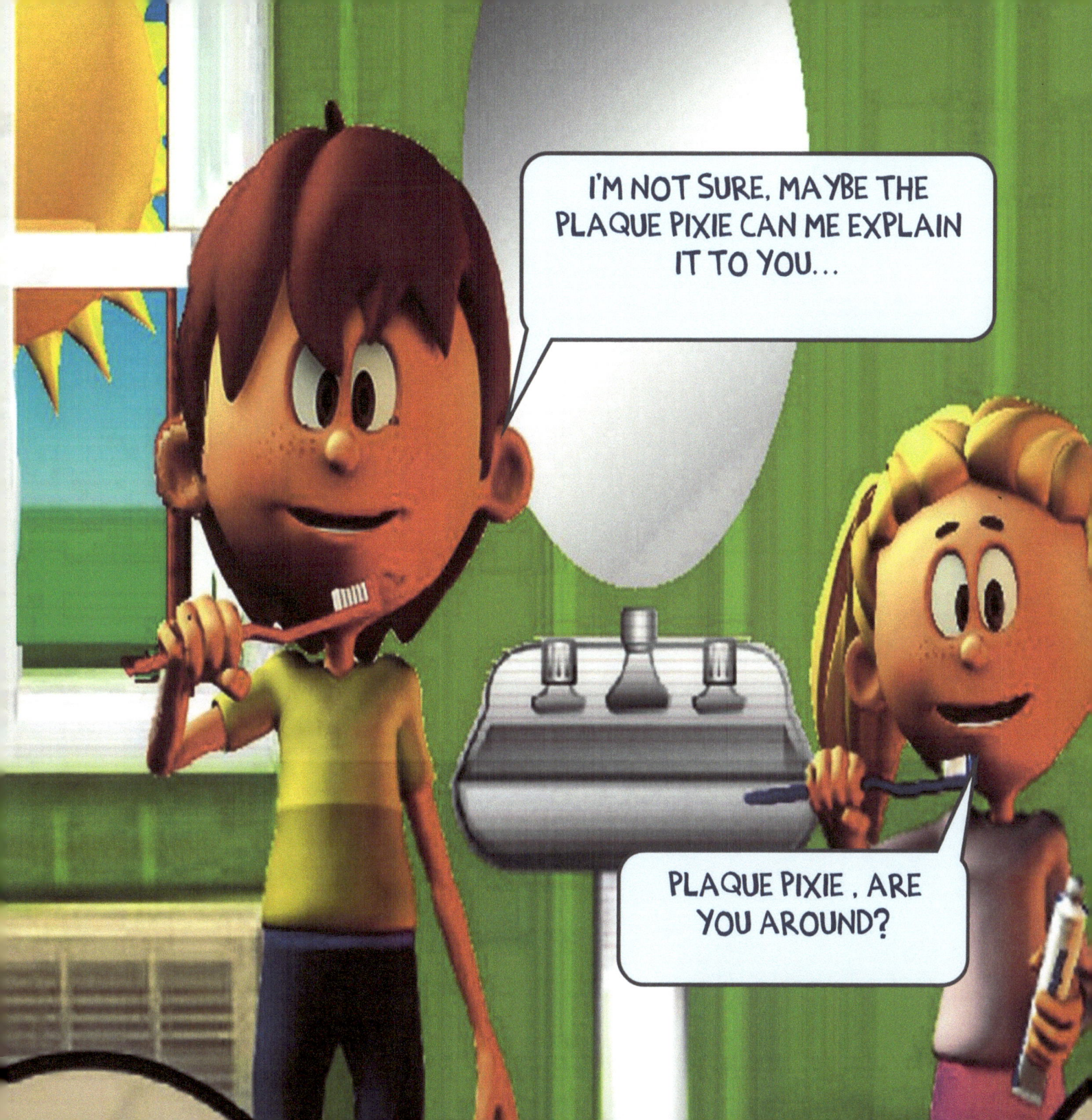

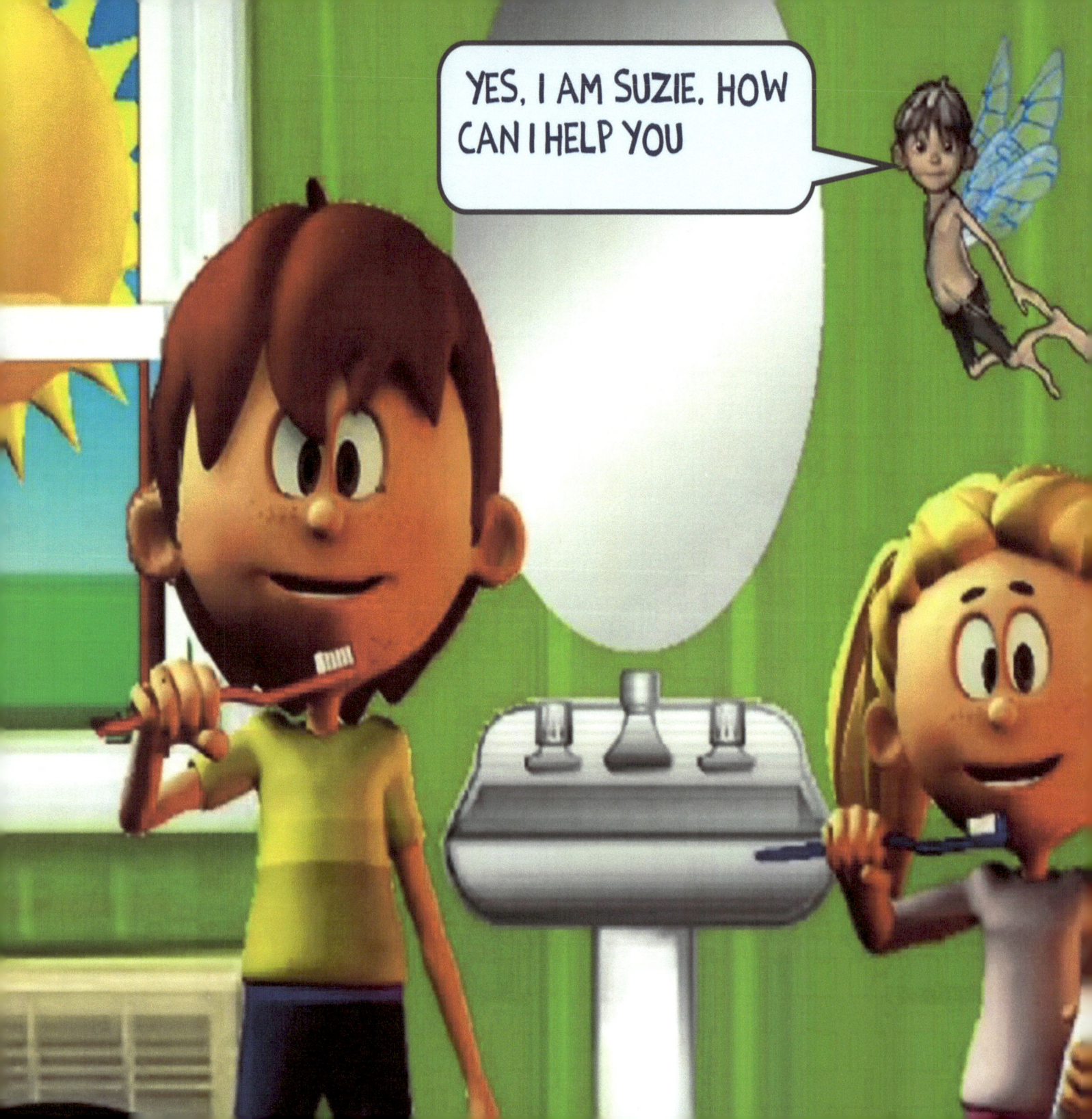

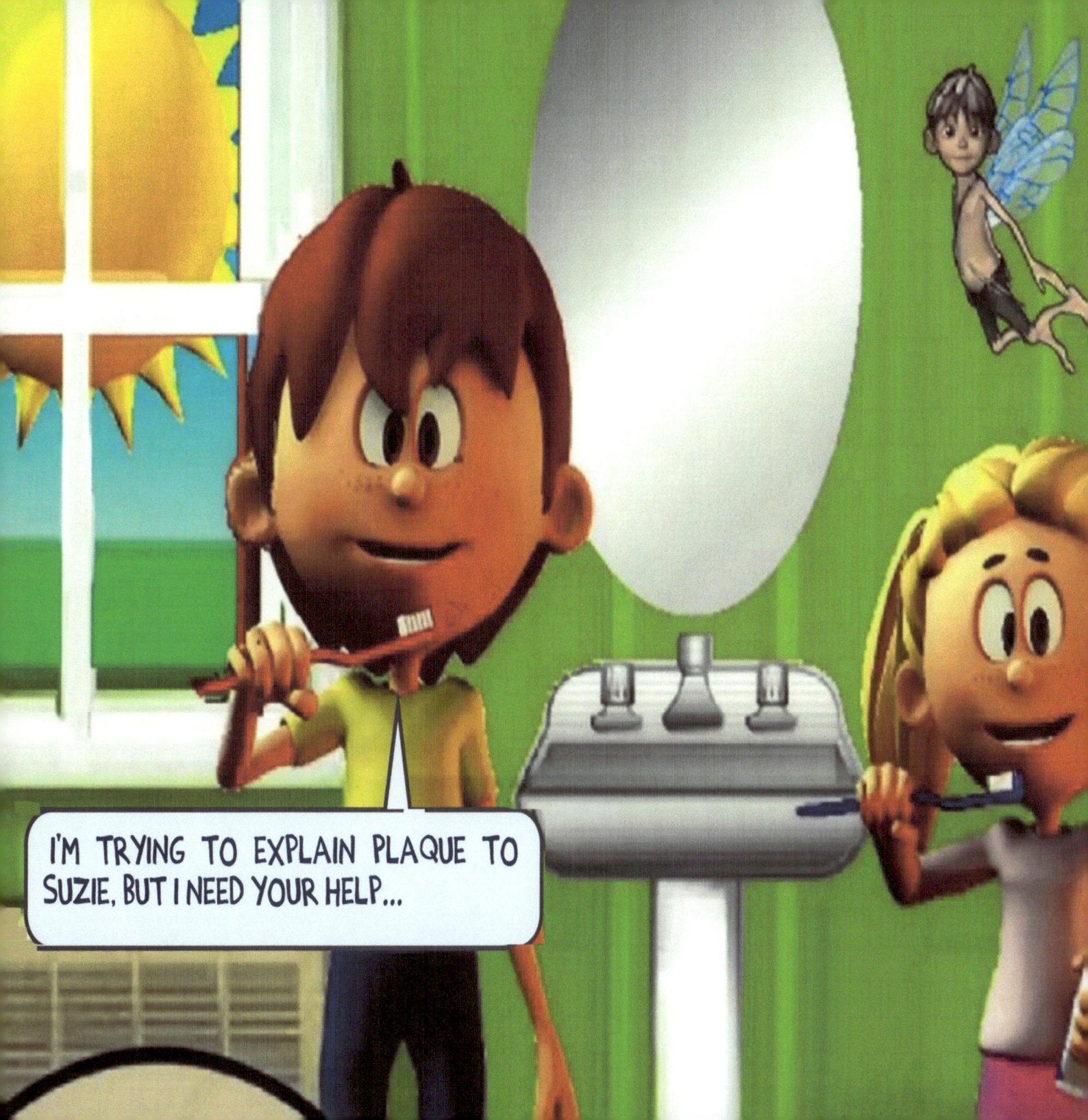

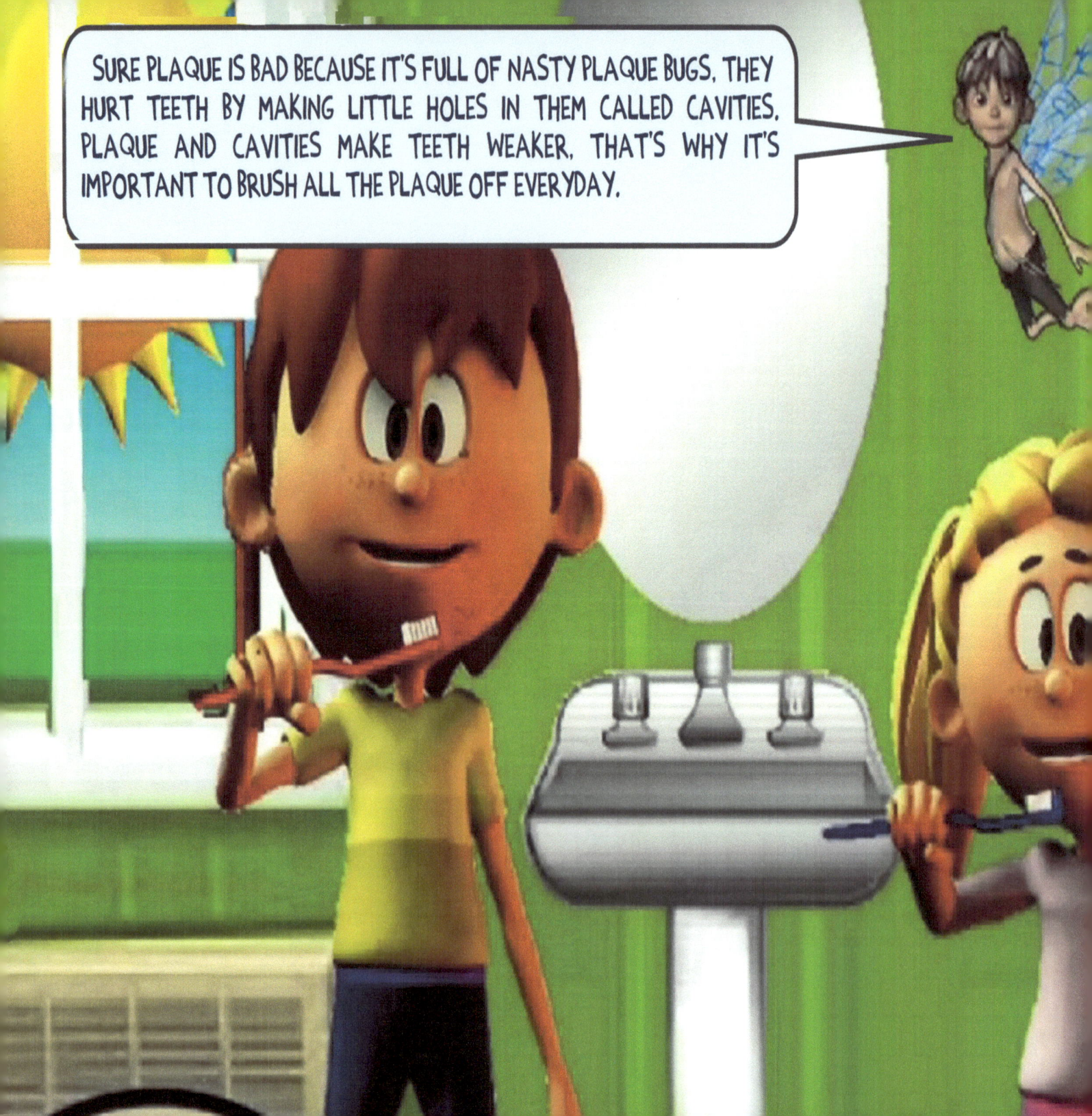

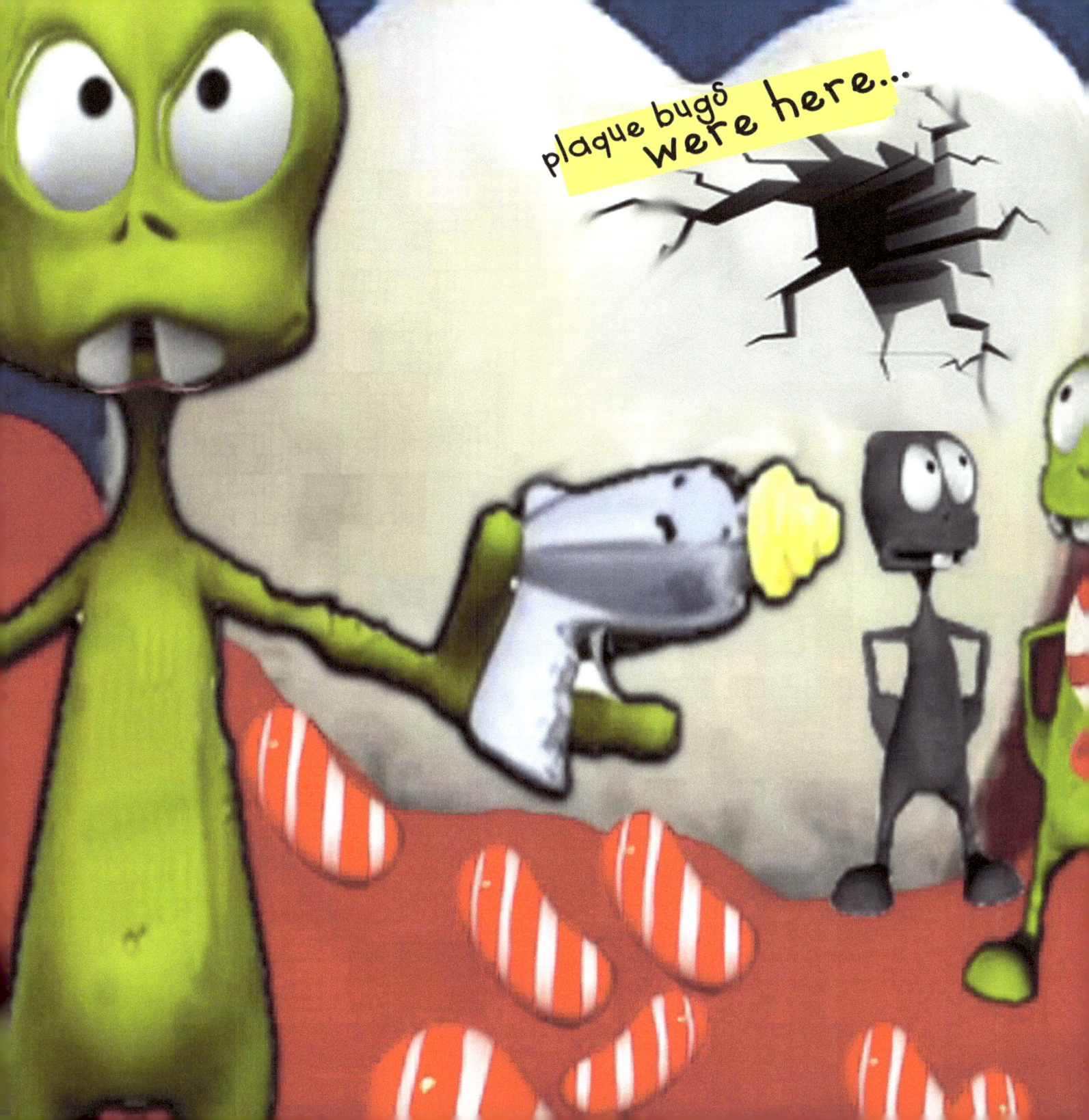

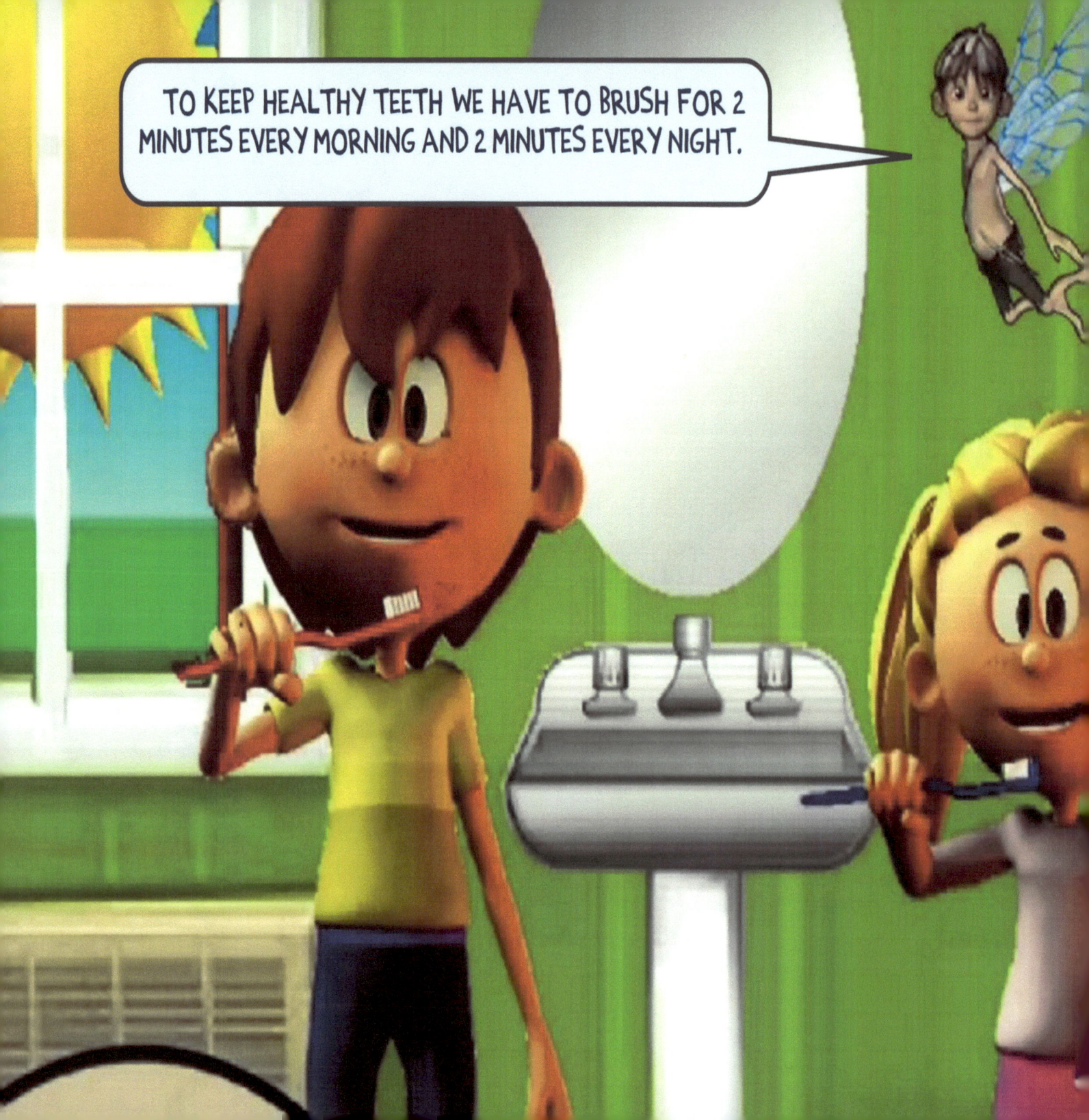

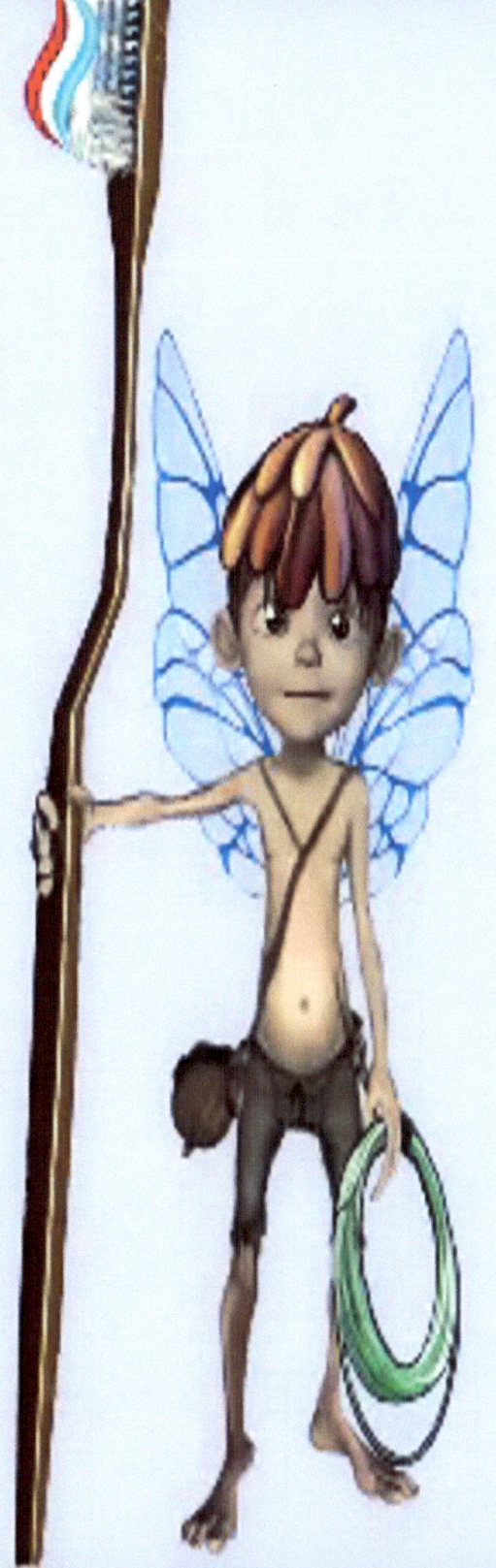

MAKE SURE TO USE A SPECIAL KIDS TOOTHBRUSH WHEN YOU BRUSH. KIDS TOOTHBRUSHES FIT LITTLE MOUTHS AND HAVE SOFT BRISTOLS.

PUT A LITTLE DOT, ABOUT THE SIZE OF A PEA OF FLUORIDE TOOTHPASTE ON THE BRUSH. ONCE YOU HAVE THE TOOTHPASTE ON THE BRUSH OPEN YOUR MOUTH WIDE. START WITH THE TEETH IN THE BACK AND BRUSH IN LITTLE CIRCLES, WORKING YOUR WAY TO THE TEETH IN THE FRONT OF YOUR MOUTH.

DON'T FORGET TO BRUSH YOUR GUMS. BRUSH THE TOP ,FRONT, AND BACK SIDES OF EACH TOOTH. MAKE SURE YOU GET THE INSIDES OF ALL THE TEETH.

WHEN YOU ARE DONE BE SURE TO SPIT OUT ALL THE TOOTHPASTE. DON'T SWALLOW THE TOOTHPASTE. IT MIGHT UPSET YOUR TUMMY.

Toothbrushing Instructions

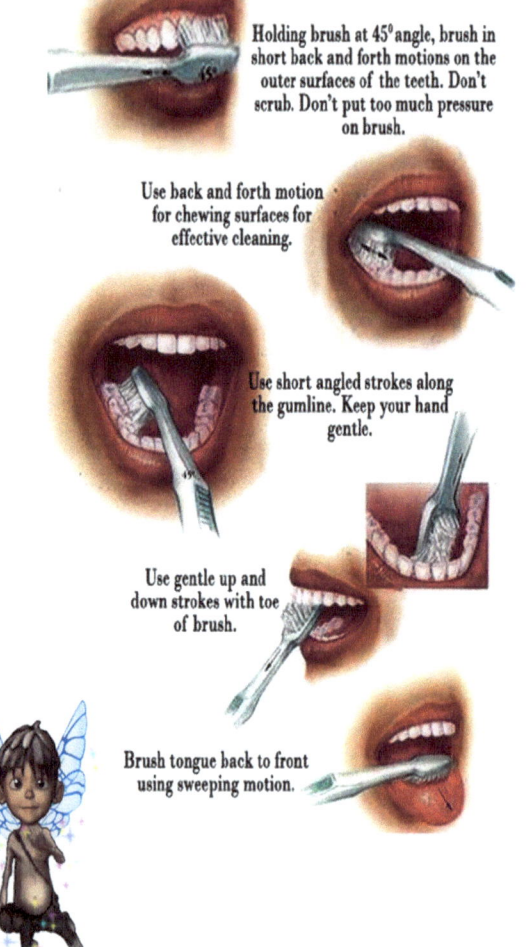

Holding brush at 45° angle, brush in short back and forth motions on the outer surfaces of the teeth. Don't scrub. Don't put too much pressure on brush.

Use back and forth motion for chewing surfaces for effective cleaning.

Use short angled strokes along the gumline. Keep your hand gentle.

Use gentle up and down strokes with toe of brush.

Brush tongue back to front using sweeping motion.

Flossing Instructions

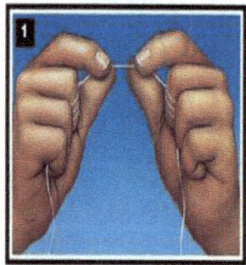

Wind 18" of floss around middle fingers of each hand. Pinch floss between thumbs and index fingers, leaving 1" - 2" length in between. Use thumbs to direct floss between upper teeth.

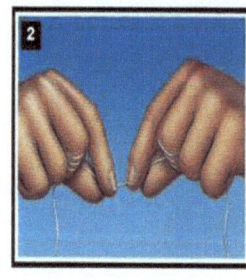

Keep a 1" - 2" length of floss taut between fingers. Use index fingers to guide floss between contacts of the lower teeth.

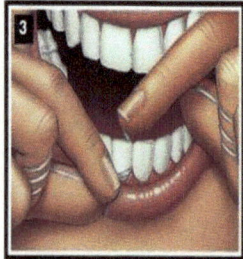

Gently guide floss between the teeth by using a zig-zag motion. DO NOT SNAP FLOSS BETWEEN YOUR TEETH. Contour floss around the side of the tooth.

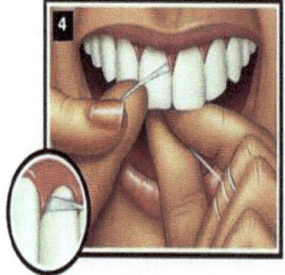

Slide floss up and down against the tooth surface and under the gumline. Floss each tooth thoroughly with a clean section of floss.

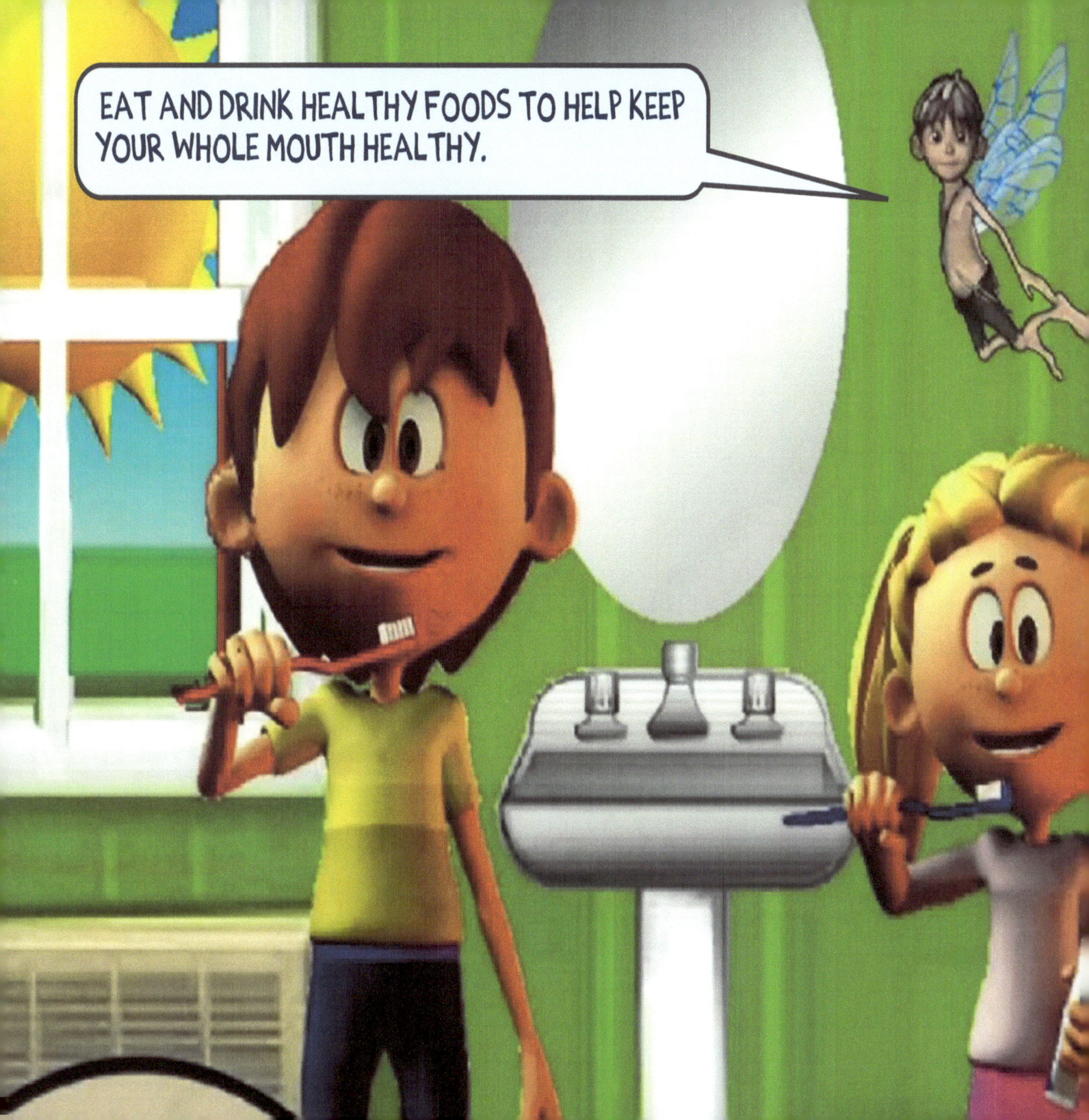

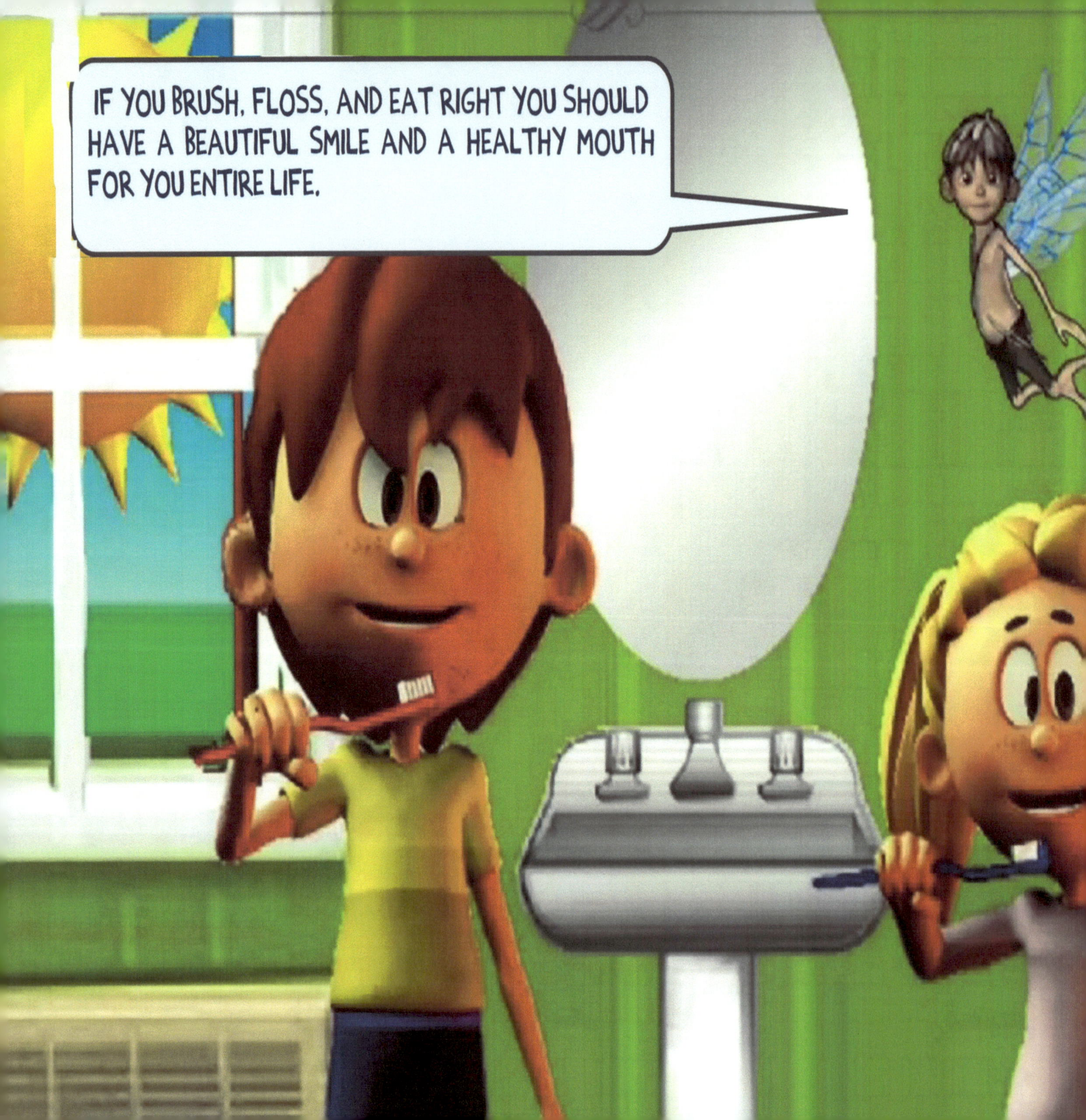

THE END

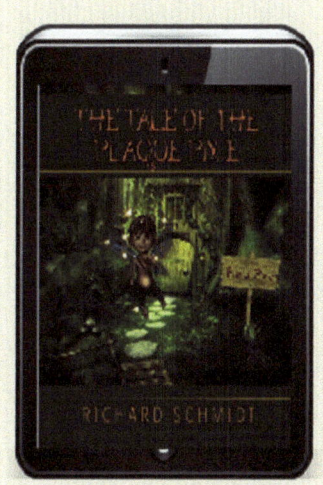
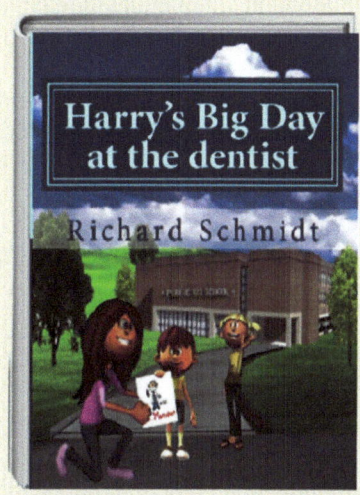